GLORIOUSTINA ESSIA

Herbal Solutions

The Comprehensive A-Z Guide to Natural Remedies for Everyday Health Concerns

Contents

INTRODUCTION

Welcome to "Herbal Solutions: The Comprehensive A-Z Guide to Natural Remedies for Everyday Health Concerns," a pivotal resource for anyone seeking to embrace the healing power of nature in addressing common health issues. This guide is a crucial companion in a world increasingly inclined towards holistic wellness, offering natural, effective alternatives for various everyday health concerns.

In these pages, we embark on a journey exploring the expansive world of herbal remedies. From the calming chamomile for sleep disturbances to the invigorating ginseng for energy boosts, this guide covers an extensive spectrum of herbs, each with unique healing properties. This encyclopedia is meticulously crafted to give you an in-depth understanding of utilizing these natural solutions effectively and safely.

The use of herbs for medicinal purposes is a tradition as old as humanity itself, deeply rooted in various cultures across the globe.

This guide is designed to be accessible to all - whether you are a seasoned herbalist, a natural medicine practitioner, or someone just beginning to explore the world of herbal remedies. Each entry in the A-Z compendium is presented in an easy-to-understand format, detailing the health concerns the herb addresses, its medicinal properties, recommended dosages, and methods of preparation.

Moreover, "Herbal Solutions" emphasizes the importance of using herbs responsibly. It includes guidance on understanding contraindications, recognizing the quality of herbal products, and navigating the nuances of herbal treatments to ensure safe and effective use. This careful consideration mirrors the growing demand for natural health solutions that are both reliable and responsibly administered.

Thus, "Herbal Solutions" is more than just a guide; it's a tool for empowerment in your health and wellness journey. It encourages you to take an active role in managing your health through natural means, fostering a deeper connection with the healing gifts of the earth. As you turn these pages, you unlock a world where health concerns are met with nature's profound solutions, leading to a harmonious balance of body, mind, and spirit.

A - COMPREHENSIVE GUIDE TO NATURAL REMEDIES FOR EVERYDAY HEALTH CONCERNS

ACNE

Acne, a common skin condition, is characterized by pimples, blackheads, and inflamed patches of skin. Herbal remedies for acne focus on anti-inflammatory and antimicrobial properties.

- **Tea Tree Oil:** Known for its antimicrobial properties. Dilute with a carrier oil and apply topically to affected areas.
- **Green Tea Extract:** Rich in antioxidants, it can be applied topically to reduce inflammation and sebum production.

ACID REFLUX

Acid reflux, or heartburn, occurs when stomach acid flows back into the oesophagus, irritating.

- **Licorice Root:** Helps to coat the stomach lining and oesophagus, reducing irritation. Use DGL (deglycyrrhizinated licorice) to avoid potential side effects.
- **Chamomile:** Soothes the digestive tract and reduces acidity. Drink a

tea after meals.

AGING

Ageing is a natural process, but certain herbal remedies can help to reduce its visible signs and improve overall vitality.

- **Ginkgo Biloba:** Improves circulation and cognitive function, often taken as a supplement.
- **Turmeric:** Its antioxidant properties help combat oxidative stress, a factor in ageing. Use in cooking or as a supplement.

ALLERGIES

Allergies occur when the immune system reacts to a foreign substance. Herbal remedies often focus on anti-inflammatory and immune-regulating properties.

- **Butterbur:** Known to reduce histamine and alleviate allergy symptoms. Take as directed, ensuring it's free of pyrrolizidine alkaloids.
- **Stinging Nettle:** Acts as a natural antihistamine. It can be taken as a tea or supplement.

ANEMIA

A lack of healthy red blood cells characterizes anaemia. Herbs high in iron and vitamins can help in managing anaemia.

- **Nettle:** High in iron, vitamins, and minerals. Consume as a tea or supplement.
- **Yellow Dock:** Known to aid in iron absorption. Best taken as a tincture or supplement.

ANXIETY

Anxiety involves persistent, excessive worry. Herbal remedies often have calming properties.

- **Valerian Root:** Acts as a natural sedative, reducing anxiety and improving sleep. Could you take it as a tea or supplement?
- **Passionflower:** Known for its calming effects, helping to alleviate nervous tension. Available in various forms, including teas and tinctures.

ARTHRITIS

Arthritis is characterized by joint pain and inflammation. Herbal treatments often focus on anti-inflammatory and analgesic properties.

- **Turmeric:** Contains curcumin, which has anti-inflammatory properties. Use in cooking or as a supplement, often combined with black pepper for absorption.
- **Ginger:** Also anti-inflammatory, it can be used in cooking, as a tea, or as a supplement.

ASTHMA

Asthma is a respiratory condition marked by spasms in the bronchi of the lungs. Herbs used for asthma often aim to reduce spasms and inflammation.

- **Licorice Root:** Has anti-inflammatory properties and acts as a bronchodilator. Use as a tea or in a tincture.
- **Mullein:** Soothes the respiratory tract. Use as a tea or inhaled as a steam.

B - COMPREHENSIVE GUIDE TO NATURAL REMEDIES FOR EVERYDAY HEALTH CONCERNS

BACK PAIN

Back pain, a common musculoskeletal complaint, can often be alleviated with herbal remedies known for their anti-inflammatory and analgesic properties.

- **Willow Bark:** Known as "nature's aspirin," it contains salicin, which reduces pain and inflammation. It can be taken as a tea or supplement.
- **Devil's Claw:** Used for its anti-inflammatory properties, it is particularly effective in lower back pain. Available in capsule form.

BAD BREATH (Halitosis)

Various factors, including dental and digestive problems, can cause bad breath. Herbal remedies focus on antibacterial and digestive health properties.

- **Peppermint:** Freshens breath and has antibacterial properties. Chew leaves or use as a mouthwash.
- **Fennel Seeds:** Natural breath freshener and aids in digestion. Chew on the seeds after meals.

BACTERIAL VAGINOSIS

Bacterial vaginosis is an imbalance of bacteria in the vagina. Herbal remedies aim to restore balance and have antibacterial properties.

- **Tea Tree Oil:** Known for its antimicrobial properties. Dilute and apply topically, but never ingest.
- **Garlic:** Natural antibiotic properties. It can be taken orally as a supplement.

BLACK EYE

A black eye is bruising around the eye due to trauma. Herbal treatments focus on reducing inflammation and speeding up healing.

- **Arnica:** Reduces swelling and promotes healing. Use as a cream or gel, but do not apply to broken skin.
- **Witch Hazel:** Acts as an astringent to reduce swelling. Apply gently with a cotton ball.

BLADDER INFECTIONS

Bladder infections, or cystitis, are typically bacterial infections. Herbal remedies aim to increase urinary tract health and have antibacterial effects.

- **Cranberry:** Prevents bacteria from adhering to the bladder walls. Available as juice or supplement.
- **Uva Ursi:** Contains compounds effective against urinary tract bacteria. Could you take it as a tea or supplement?

BLEEDING DISORDERS

Bleeding disorders affect the body's ability to clot blood. Herbs used are those known for their hemostatic properties.

- **Yarrow:** Known to stop bleeding and is anti-inflammatory. It can be used topically or taken as a tea.
- **Nettle:** Rich in vitamin K, which is crucial for blood clotting. Consume as tea or in cooked dishes.

BLOOD CLOTS

Blood clots can be dangerous and require medical attention. Certain herbs are known for their blood-thinning properties.

- **Ginkgo Biloba:** Helps improve blood circulation and has blood-thinning effects. Usually taken as a supplement.
- **Garlic:** Known to reduce blood clotting. Include in diet or take as a supplement.

BOILS

Boils are painful, pus-filled bumps under the skin caused by bacterial infections. Herbal remedies focus on antibacterial and anti-inflammatory properties.

- **Turmeric:** Apply a paste of turmeric and water to the boil for its antibacterial properties.
- **Tea Tree Oil:** Apply diluted oil to the boil for its antimicrobial effects.

BRUISES

Bruises are caused by blood vessels breaking under the skin. Herbal remedies can help speed up healing and reduce swelling.

- **Arnica:** Known to reduce swelling and speed up healing. Apply as a cream or gel.
- **Comfrey:** Has skin-healing properties. Use in a poultice or as a cream.

Herbal remedies can effectively treat these conditions, but it's important to remember that they are not substitutes for professional medical advice, especially in serious conditions like blood clots. Consulting with a healthcare professional before starting any new treatment is always recommended.

C – COMPREHENSIVE GUIDE TO NATURAL REMEDIES FOR EVERYDAY HEALTH CONCERNS

CHICKENPOX

Chickenpox, a viral infection characterized by itchy, red blisters, can be managed with herbs known for their soothing and anti-inflammatory properties.

- **Oatmeal Bath:** Oatmeal has soothing properties that relieve itching. Use colloidal oatmeal in baths.
- **Calendula Cream:** Helps in healing blisters and reducing inflammation. Apply topically on non-broken skin areas.

CHLAMYDIA

Chlamydia is a bacterial infection requiring medical treatment. Certain herbs may assist in complementing traditional antibiotic therapy.

- **Goldenseal:** Known for its antimicrobial properties. Take it as a supplement or tea.
- **Garlic:** Has natural antibiotic effects. Include in diet or take as a supplement.

CHOLERA

Cholera, a severe diarrheal illness, requires immediate medical attention. Some herbs can aid hydration and recovery post-infection.

- **Ginger Tea:** Helps in settling the stomach and reducing nausea. Drink ginger tea in small amounts.
- **Cinnamon:** Has antimicrobial properties and can be soothing for the digestive system. Add to teas or foods.

CHRONIC FATIGUE SYNDROME

Chronic Fatigue Syndrome (CFS) is characterized by extreme tiredness. Herbs that boost energy and improve overall vitality can be beneficial.

- **Ginseng:** Known for boosting energy and endurance. Take it as a supplement or tea.
- **Ashwagandha:** An adaptogen that helps in managing stress and improving energy levels. Available in supplement form.

COLD SORES

Cold sores, caused by the herpes simplex virus, appear as blisters around the mouth. Herbal treatments focus on antiviral properties.

- **Lemon Balm:** Known for its antiviral properties against herpes simplex virus. Apply as a cream to the affected area.
- **Tea Tree Oil:** Apply diluted oil to the sore for its antiviral effects.

COMMON COLD

The common cold, a viral respiratory infection, can be managed with herbs that boost immunity and relieve symptoms.

- **Echinacea:** Boosts the immune system and can reduce the duration of a cold. Take it as a tea or supplement.
- **Elderberry:** Has antiviral properties and can alleviate cold symptoms. Consume as syrup or tablets.

CONJUNCTIVITIS (Pink Eye)

Conjunctivitis is an inflammation of the eye's outer membrane. Herbal remedies can be used for soothing relief.

- **Chamomile:** Anti-inflammatory properties can soothe irritation. Use as a warm compress (ensure it's sterile).
- **Eyebright (Euphrasia):** Traditionally used for eye irritations. Use as a sterile eye wash.

CONSTIPATION

Constipation can be relieved with herbs that have laxative properties and aid in digestion.

- **Psyllium Husk:** A natural fibre that helps in bowel movement. Take it with plenty of water.
- **Senna:** A strong herbal laxative. Use sparingly and only as needed.

COUGH

Herbal remedies for coughs aim to soothe the throat and loosen mucus.

- **Thyme:** Helps relieve cough and loosens phlegm. Use as a tea or in syrup.
- **Licorice Root:** Soothes the throat and helps with coughs. Drink as tea or use in cough syrups.

D - COMPREHENSIVE GUIDE TO NATURAL REMEDIES FOR EVERYDAY HEALTH CONCERNS

DANDRUFF

Dandruff is characterized by flaking and itching of the scalp and can be managed using herbal remedies with antifungal and soothing properties.

- **Tea Tree Oil:** Known for its antifungal properties. Add a few drops to shampoo or apply diluted oil directly to the scalp.
- **Aloe Vera:** Soothes the scalp and reduces irritation. Apply aloe vera gel directly to the scalp.

DEHYDRATION

Dehydration occurs when the body loses more fluids than it takes in. Herbal remedies can aid in rehydration and maintaining fluid balance.

- **Chamomile Tea:** Mildly hydrating and soothing for the digestive system. It can be consumed as a gentle rehydrating beverage.
- **Ginger Tea:** Helps in rehydration, especially after nausea or vomiting. Drink in moderation.

DEPRESSION

Depression is a mood disorder requiring professional treatment. Some herbs are known for their mood-boosting and antidepressant properties.

- **St. John's Wort:** Widely used for mild to moderate depression. Consult a healthcare provider before use, especially if on other medications.
- **Saffron:** Has shown promise in clinical studies for treating mild to moderate depression. Use as a spice in food or as a supplement.

DIABETES

Diabetes is a chronic condition affecting blood sugar regulation. Some herbs can help manage blood sugar levels.

- **Cinnamon:** Known to help lower blood sugar levels. Add to foods or take as a supplement.
- **Fenugreek:** Seeds are beneficial in controlling blood sugar. It can be consumed as seeds, in food, or as a supplement.

DIARRHEA

Diarrhea involves frequent, loose bowel movements. Herbal remedies can aid in solidifying stool and soothing the digestive tract.

- **Slippery Elm:** Forms a soothing gel that coats the lining of the digestive tract. Consume as a tea or in capsules.
- **Blackberry and Raspberry Leaves** Contain tannins that help tighten the gut lining. Drink as a tea.

DRY EYE SYNDROME

Dry eye syndrome involves dry, uncomfortable eyes. Certain herbs can help in alleviating these symptoms.

- **Chamomile:** Anti-inflammatory properties can soothe dry eyes. Use as a warm compress (make sure it's sterile).
- **Eyebright:** Traditionally used for eye health. Use as a sterile eye wash or in compresses.

DYSENTERY

Dysentery, a severe form of diarrhea with blood, requires medical attention. Some herbs can support recovery.

- **Goldenseal:** Has antimicrobial properties. Take it as a supplement or tea, but consult a healthcare professional first.
- **Aloe Vera Juice:** Soothing to the digestive tract can help heal. Drink pure aloe vera juice in small quantities.

Digestive Health

In natural wellness, digestive health is a cornerstone, profoundly influencing overall well-being. This chapter delves into herbal remedies used traditionally and validated by modern research to support and enhance digestive health.

Understanding Digestive Health

Digestive health is pivotal to our overall well-being. A healthy digestive system processes food, absorbs essential nutrients, and plays a crucial role in immunity. Common digestive issues include indigestion, acid reflux, bloating, constipation, and diarrhea, which can often be effectively managed with herbal remedies.

Herbal Remedies for Common Digestive Problems

Ginger (Zingiber officinale)

- **Uses:** Eases nausea, stimulates digestion, and combats motion sickness.
- **How to Use:** Ginger can be consumed as tea, in capsules, or as fresh or dried root in cooking.

Peppermint (Mentha piperita)

- **Uses:** Alleviates irritable bowel syndrome (IBS) symptoms, including bloating and intestinal spasms.
- **How to Use:** Often taken as enteric-coated capsules, tea, or oil in small doses.

Chamomile (Matricaria chamomilla)

- **Uses:** Soothes stomach aches and relieves diarrhoea. It also has calming effects that can help with stress-related digestive issues.
- **How to Use:** Commonly consumed as a gentle, calming tea.

Licorice Root (Glycyrrhiza glabra)

- **Uses:** Treats acid reflux and ulcers; has anti-inflammatory properties.
- **How to Use:** Available as DGL (deglycyrrhizinated licorice) tablets, tea, or powder.

Fennel (Foeniculum vulgare)

- **Uses:** Reduces gas and bloating, aids digestion, and can ease infant colic.
- **How to Use:** It can be chewed as seeds, brewed as tea, or taken as supplements.

Integrating Herbs into Daily Diet

Incorporating these herbs into your daily diet can be a simple and effective way to improve digestive health. Adding ginger to meals, drinking a cup of peppermint or chamomile tea after dinner, or using fennel seeds in cooking are practical ways to enjoy the digestive benefits of these herbs.

Safety and Considerations

While herbal remedies are generally safe, it's important to consider potential interactions with medications and individual allergies. Pregnant or breast-feeding women and individuals with chronic health conditions should consult with healthcare professionals before starting any herbal regimen.

E - COMPREHENSIVE GUIDE TO NATURAL REMEDIES FOR EVERYDAY HEALTH CONCERNS

EAR INFECTIONS

Ear infections, often characterized by pain and inflammation, can sometimes be managed with herbal remedies known for their antimicrobial and soothing properties.

- **Garlic Oil:** Known for its antibacterial and antiviral properties. Apply warm garlic oil drops into the ear, but avoid if the eardrum is perforated.
- **Mullein Drops:** Often combined with garlic oil, mullein can reduce inflammation. Use as ear drops, ensuring there's no eardrum perforation.

EATING DISORDERS

Eating disorders are serious conditions that require professional treatment. Herbs may support recovery by promoting a healthy appetite and stress relief.

- **Peppermint:** Can stimulate appetite and aid digestion. Drink as a tea.
- **Chamomile:** Has calming properties, beneficial for stress and anxiety often associated with eating disorders. Consume as a tea.

ECZEMA

Eczema, a condition causing itchy, inflamed skin, can be alleviated with herbs known for their anti-inflammatory and soothing properties.

- **Chamomile Cream:** Soothes and reduces inflammation in the skin. Use topically as a cream or lotion.
- **Calendula:** Promotes healing and soothes eczema. Apply as a cream or ointment.

EDEMA

Edema, the swelling caused by excess fluid trapped in the body's tissues, can be managed with diuretic herbs that help reduce fluid retention.

- **Dandelion:** Acts as a natural diuretic. Consume as a tea or supplement.
- **Parsley:** Another natural diuretic. Use fresh ingredients in foods or as tea.

EMPHYSEMA

Emphysema, a chronic lung condition, is best managed under medical supervision. Certain herbs can support lung health.

- **Lobelia:** Thought to help relax the airways and ease breathing. Use with caution and under professional advice.
- **Gingko Biloba:** Improves circulation and lung function. Take it as a supplement.

ENDOMETRIOSIS

Endometriosis involves painful tissues outside the uterus. Herbs can be used to manage symptoms like pain and inflammation.

- **Turmeric:** Contains curcumin, which helps reduce inflammation. Use in cooking or as a supplement.
- **Ginger:** Reduces inflammation and can alleviate pain. Drink as tea or use in cooking.

ERECTILE DYSFUNCTION

Erectile dysfunction can often be a symptom of underlying health issues. Some herbs are known to help improve circulation and libido.

- **Ginseng:** Shown to improve erectile function. Take it as a supplement.
- **Horny Goat Weed:** Has a long history of use for improving sexual function. Take as directed in supplement form.

F - COMPREHENSIVE GUIDE TO NATURAL REMEDIES FOR EVERYDAY HEALTH CONCERNS

FATIGUE

Fatigue, a common symptom characterized by a chronic state of tiredness, can be managed using herbs known for their energizing and adaptogenic properties.

- **Ashwagandha:** An adaptogen that helps the body resist stressors and combat fatigue. Take it as a supplement or in powder form.
- **Rhodiola Rosea:** Known for increasing energy, stamina, and mental capacity. Use as directed in supplement form.

FIBROMYALGIA

Fibromyalgia, a condition marked by widespread pain and fatigue, can benefit from herbs that have pain-relieving and anti-inflammatory properties.

- **Turmeric:** Contains curcumin, which has anti-inflammatory effects. Use in cooking or as a supplement.
- **St. John's Wort:** Has nerve pain-relieving properties. Take it as a tea, tincture, or supplement.

FLATULENCE

Flatulence or gas can be embarrassing and uncomfortable. Certain herbs can aid in digestion and reduce gas production.

- **Fennel Seeds:** Help in reducing bloating and gas. Chew fennel seeds after meals or drink as tea.
- **Peppermint:** Relieves intestinal spasms and gas. Drink as a tea or take enteric-coated capsules.

FOOD POISONING

Food poisoning, typically caused by bacteria, viruses, or parasites in contaminated food, can be alleviated with herbs known for their antimicrobial properties.

- **Ginger:** Helps to settle the stomach and reduce nausea. Drink as a tea.
- **Activated Charcoal:** Not an herb, but a natural remedy used to absorb toxins. Take as directed after consulting with a healthcare professional.

FRACTURES

While fractures require medical treatment and proper immobilization, some herbs can support bone healing.

- **Comfrey:** Known for its bone and tissue healing properties. Use as a poultice or cream for external application around the fractured area (not on open wounds).
- **Horsetail:** Rich in silica, which is essential for bone repair. Take as a tea or supplement, but under professional guidance.

G - COMPREHENSIVE GUIDE TO NATURAL REMEDIES FOR EVERYDAY HEALTH CONCERNS

GALLSTONES

Gallstones are hardened deposits in the gallbladder that can cause pain and digestive problems. Certain herbs can help manage the symptoms and prevent new stone formation.

- **Milk Thistle:** Known for supporting liver and gallbladder health. It helps in bile flow, which can reduce the risk of gallstones. Available as a supplement or tea.
- **Dandelion:** Acts as a liver tonic and may help in bile flow. Use it as a tea or a supplement, but avoid it if you have an obstructed bile duct.

GENITAL HERPES

Genital herpes, a sexually transmitted infection caused by the herpes simplex virus, can be managed with antiviral herbs to reduce the frequency and severity of outbreaks.

- **Lemon Balm:** Known for its antiviral properties against herpes simplex virus. Apply lemon balm cream to the affected area.

- **Echinacea:** Can boost the immune system and potentially reduce the frequency of herpes flare-ups. Take it as a tea or supplement.

GENITAL WARTS

Genital warts are caused by certain strains of the human papillomavirus (HPV). Herbal treatments can be used alongside conventional treatments to help clear the warts.

- **Tea Tree Oil:** Has antiviral properties. Apply diluted tea tree oil to the warts, but use it cautiously due to its potency and potential skin irritation.
- **Green Tea Extract:** A specific formulation of green tea extract, known as sinecatechins (Veregen), is FDA-approved for treating genital warts. Apply as directed.

GUM DISEASE

Gum disease, or periodontitis, is an infection of the gums that can lead to tooth loss. Herbal remedies can help maintain oral health and treat mild gum disease.

- **Aloe Vera Gel:** Known for its anti-inflammatory and healing properties. Apply directly to the gums or use it as a mouthwash.
- **Clove Oil:** Effective for reducing gum inflammation and pain due to its eugenol content. Apply diluted clove oil to the gums or use it in a mouth rinse.

H - COMPREHENSIVE GUIDE TO NATURAL REMEDIES FOR EVERYDAY HEALTH CONCERNS

HAIR LOSS

Hair loss can be due to various factors, including genetics, stress, and hormonal imbalances. Herbal remedies can help in promoting hair growth and maintaining scalp health.

- **Saw Palmetto:** Believed to slow hair loss and stimulate hair growth. Use as a supplement.
- **Rosemary Oil:** Applied topically, it can stimulate hair growth and improve scalp circulation.

HALITOSIS (Bad Breath)

Halitosis, or bad breath, often originates from oral or digestive issues. Herbs with antimicrobial and digestive properties can help.

- **Peppermint:** Freshens breath and has antibacterial properties. Chew leaves or use as a mouthwash.
- **Fennel Seeds:** Natural breath freshener and aids in digestion. Chew on the seeds after meals.

HEADACHES

Headaches, including migraines, can be alleviated using herbs with pain-relieving and anti-inflammatory properties.

- **Feverfew:** Known to reduce the frequency and severity of migraines. Take it as a supplement.
- **Lavender Oil:** Inhaling lavender oil can help relieve migraine pain. Use in aromatherapy.

HEART DISEASE

While medical supervision is crucial for heart disease, certain herbs can support heart health.

- **Hawthorn:** Known for its heart-protective properties. It can improve cardiac function and circulation. Take it as a tea or supplement.
- **Garlic:** Helps in lowering blood pressure and cholesterol levels. Include in diet or take as a supplement.

HEMORRHOIDS

Hemorrhoids are swollen veins in the lower rectum and anus, often causing discomfort. Herbs with anti-inflammatory properties can provide relief.

- **Witch Hazel:** Applied topically, it can reduce itching and swelling. Use as a cream or ointment.
- **Horse Chestnut:** Helps in reducing inflammation and swelling. Take as a supplement, but not to be applied directly to hemorrhoids.

HEPATITIS

Hepatitis, inflammation of the liver, requires medical attention. Certain herbs can support liver health.

- **Milk Thistle:** Known for its liver-protective qualities. Helps in liver detoxification. Available as a supplement.
- **Dandelion Root:** Acts as a liver tonic and helps in bile flow. Drink as a tea.

HERPES SIMPLEX

Herpes simplex is a viral infection. Antiviral herbs can help manage outbreaks.

- **Lemon Balm:** Known for its antiviral properties against herpes simplex virus. Apply as a cream or use in tea.
- **Licorice Root:** Contains glycyrrhizin, which has antiviral properties. Use as a tea, cream, or supplement.

HIGH BLOOD PRESSURE

Herbs that promote relaxation and vascular health can aid in managing high blood pressure.

- **Hibiscus Tea:** Can lower blood pressure. Drink 1-2 cups of hibiscus tea daily.
- **Garlic:** Helps in lowering blood pressure. Include in diet or take as a supplement.

HIGH CHOLESTEROL

Herbal remedies can assist in managing cholesterol levels.

- **Red Yeast Rice** Contains compounds similar to statins, which can help lower cholesterol. Take it as a supplement, but consult a doctor first.
- **Artichoke Leaf Extract:** Helps in lowering LDL (bad) cholesterol. Available as a supplement.

HIVES

Hives, or urticaria, are an allergic reaction causing itchy welts. Herbs with antihistamine properties can provide relief.

- **Nettle:** Acts as a natural antihistamine. Take it as a tea or supplement.
- **Chamomile:** Known for its anti-inflammatory and soothing properties, which can help alleviate the itchiness of hives. Use as a tea or apply topically as a cream or lotion.

HOT FLASHES

Hot flashes, common during menopause, can be managed using herbs that have natural phytoestrogen properties or help regulate body temperature.

- **Black Cohosh:** Often used to reduce menopausal symptoms like hot flashes. Take it as a supplement.
- **Red Clover:** Contains isoflavones, which are plant-based estrogens. It may help balance hormones and reduce hot flashes. Available as teas or supplements.

I - COMPREHENSIVE GUIDE TO NATURAL REMEDIES FOR EVERYDAY HEALTH CONCERNS

IMPOTENCE (Erectile Dysfunction)

Impotence, or erectile dysfunction, is a common problem that can stem from various causes, including psychological and physical factors. Some herbs are known to help improve circulation and enhance libido.

- **Ginseng:** Particularly Panax ginseng has shown promise in improving erectile function. Take it as a supplement.
- **Horny Goat Weed:** Traditionally used for erectile dysfunction and low libido. Use as directed in supplement form.

INCONTINENCE

Urinary incontinence involves a loss of bladder control. Certain herbs can strengthen the bladder and pelvic muscles.

- **Saw Palmetto:** This may be beneficial for men with prostate-induced incontinence. Take it as a supplement.
- **Horsetail:** Known for its astringent properties, it can tone the bladder. Take it as a tea or supplement.

INDIGESTION

Indigestion, or dyspepsia, is a common digestive issue. Herbs can aid in soothing the stomach and improving digestion.

- **Peppermint:** Relieves indigestion and irritable bowel syndrome symptoms. Drink as a tea or take enteric-coated capsules.
- **Ginger:** Helps settle the stomach and promotes digestion. Drink it as tea or use it fresh in cooking.

INFLUENZA (Flu)

Influenza, a viral infection, can be managed with herbs known for their antiviral and immune-boosting properties.

- **Elderberry:** Known for its antiviral properties against flu viruses. Consume as syrup or tablets.
- **Echinacea:** Boosts the immune system and may reduce the duration of the flu. Take it as a tea, tincture, or supplement.

INGROWN TOENAILS

Ingrown toenails can cause pain and infection. Herbal remedies can soothe inflammation and prevent infection.

- **Tea Tree Oil:** Apply diluted tea tree oil to the affected area for its antiseptic properties.
- **Epsom Salt:** Not an herb but a natural remedy. Soak feet in Epsom salt water to reduce pain and swelling.

INSOMNIA

Insomnia involves difficulty falling or staying asleep. Herbal remedies can help induce relaxation and sleep.

- **Valerian Root:** Acts as a natural sedative. Take it as a supplement or tea before bedtime.
- **Lavender:** Inhaling or using lavender oil in a diffuser can promote relaxation and improve sleep quality.

IRRITABLE BOWEL SYNDROME (IBS)

IBS is a common gastrointestinal disorder causing pain, bloating, constipation, and diarrhea. Certain herbs can help manage symptoms.

- **Peppermint Oil:** Known to relieve IBS symptoms, especially abdominal pain and bloating. Take enteric-coated capsules to target the intestines.
- **Fennel Seeds:** Help in reducing bloating and spasms. Chew fennel seeds or drink them as tea.

Immune Support and Prevention

In pursuing health and longevity, bolstering the immune system is key.

Understanding the Immune System

The immune system is our body's defense mechanism against infections and diseases. A strong immune system fights off pathogens and maintains overall health and vitality. Factors like stress, poor diet, lack of sleep, and environmental toxins can weaken it, making the body more susceptible to illnesses.

Herbal Remedies for Immune Support

Echinacea (Echinacea spp.)

- **Uses:** Enhances the immune system and reduces the severity and duration of colds and other upper respiratory infections.
- **How to Use:** Available in teas, capsules, tinctures, and topical applications.

Elderberry (Sambucus nigra)

- **Uses:** Known for its antiviral properties, it is particularly effective against flu viruses.
- **How to Use:** Often consumed as syrup, tablets, or capsules.

Astragalus (Astragalus membranaceus)

- **Uses:** Boosts the immune system and has antioxidant properties that protect cells from damage.
- **How to Use:** Typically taken as a supplement, in tinctures, or added to soups.

Garlic (Allium sativum)

- **Uses:** Has antimicrobial and antiviral properties and is known to enhance immune function.
- **How to Use:** It can be eaten raw, cooked in dishes, or taken as supplements.

Turmeric (Curcuma longa)

- **Uses:** Contains curcumin, which has anti-inflammatory and immune-boosting properties.

- **How to Use:** Commonly used in cooking or as a supplement. Often combined with black pepper to enhance absorption.

Incorporating Herbs for Immune Health

Integrating these herbs into daily routines can significantly bolster the immune system. From adding garlic to meals to enjoying a cup of Echinacea tea to taking an Astragalus supplement, these simple practices can fortify the body's defences.

Safety and Considerations

While herbal remedies can be highly beneficial for immune support, they should be used judiciously. Some herbs can interact with medications, and individuals with autoimmune diseases or immunosuppressive therapy need to consult healthcare professionals before using these herbs.

J - COMPREHENSIVE GUIDE TO NATURAL REMEDIES FOR EVERYDAY HEALTH CONCERNS

JAUNDICE

Jaundice, characterized by yellowing of the skin and eyes, is often a symptom of liver dysfunction. Herbal remedies can support liver health and aid in the treatment of jaundice.

- **Milk Thistle:** Known for its liver-protective qualities. Helps in liver detoxification and is beneficial in treating jaundice. Available as a supplement or tea.
- **Dandelion:** Acts as a liver tonic, promoting bile flow and improving liver function. Drink as a tea or use as a supplement.

JET LAG

Jet lag occurs due to rapid travel across time zones, disrupting the body's internal clock. Herbs that help regulate sleep patterns and reduce fatigue can be beneficial.

- **Melatonin:** While not an herb, melatonin supplements can help reset the body's internal clock. Take as directed for short-term relief.

- **Valerian Root:** Known to improve sleep quality and help adjust sleep cycles. Take it as a tea or supplement upon arrival at your destination.

JOINT PAIN

Joint pain, often due to arthritis or other inflammatory conditions, can be relieved with herbs known for their anti-inflammatory and pain-relieving properties.

- **Turmeric:** Contains curcumin, which has potent anti-inflammatory effects. Use in cooking or as a supplement, often combined with black pepper for better absorption.
- **Ginger** Also has anti-inflammatory properties and can reduce joint pain. Use fresh in cooking, as a tea, or as a supplement.

K - COMPREHENSIVE GUIDE TO NATURAL REMEDIES FOR EVERYDAY HEALTH CONCERNS

KIDNEY DISEASE

Kidney disease involves the gradual loss of kidney function. Herbs used in this context can support kidney health and help manage symptoms, but using them under medical supervision is crucial, as some herbs can harm kidney disease.

- **Nettle Leaf:** Acts as a natural diuretic and kidney tonic. It can help in managing symptoms of kidney disease. Use as a tea, but consult a healthcare provider first.
- **Dandelion Root:** Known for its diuretic properties and support of kidney function. Consume as tea or a supplement, with medical guidance.

KIDNEY STONES

Kidney stones are hard mineral deposits formed in the kidneys. Certain herbs can aid in preventing stone formation and alleviating symptoms.

- **Chanca Piedra:** Known as a "stone breaker," it's traditionally used to help dissolve kidney stones. Take it as a tea or supplement.

- **Hydrangea Root:** Used historically for kidney health and may help break down kidney stones. Consume as a tea or supplement under healthcare supervision.

Managing kidney-related conditions with herbs requires caution. While certain herbs can support kidney function and help in the case of kidney stones, they should never replace conventional medical treatment, especially in serious cases of kidney disease. It's important to consult with a healthcare professional before starting any herbal remedy, particularly for individuals with kidney disease, to ensure safety and proper treatment.

L - COMPREHENSIVE GUIDE TO NATURAL REMEDIES FOR EVERYDAY HEALTH CONCERNS

LACTOSE INTOLERANCE

Lactose intolerance is the inability to digest lactose, a sugar in milk and dairy products. Herbal remedies can help in managing digestive symptoms.

- **Peppermint:** Relieves gastrointestinal symptoms like bloating and gas. Drink as a tea after meals.
- **Ginger:** Aids in digestion and can alleviate stomach discomfort. Use fresh ginger in cooking or drink as a tea.

LEUKEMIA

Leukemia, a cancer affecting blood cells, requires conventional medical treatment. Certain herbs may support overall health and complement cancer treatments.

- **Green Tea:** Rich in antioxidants, it may have anti-cancer properties. Drink as a tea, but discuss with an oncologist before use, as it can interact with certain cancer medications.
- **Astragalus:** Used in Traditional Chinese Medicine to support immune

function, which can be beneficial during cancer treatments. Take it as a supplement or tea under medical guidance.

LIVER DISEASE

Liver disease covers a range of conditions affecting liver function. Herbs can support liver health and aid in detoxification.

- **Milk Thistle:** Known for its liver-protective effects. Helps detoxify the liver and improve liver function. Available as a supplement or tea.
- **Dandelion Root:** Acts as a liver tonic and promotes bile flow. Drink as a tea or use as a supplement.

LOW BACK PAIN

Low back pain is a common ailment that can often be managed with natural remedies known for their anti-inflammatory and pain-relieving properties.

- **Devil's Claw:** Known for its anti-inflammatory properties and can help reduce back pain. Take it as a supplement.
- **Willow Bark:** Often called "nature's aspirin," it has pain-relieving properties. Use as a tea or supplement.

LOW BLOOD PRESSURE (Hypotension)

Low blood pressure can cause dizziness and fainting. Herbs that help in regulating blood pressure and improving circulation can be beneficial.

- **Licorice Root:** Can help elevate blood pressure levels. Take it cautiously as a tea or supplement, as it can interact with certain medications and conditions.
- **Ginger:** Improves circulation and can help in managing low blood pressure symptoms. Use in cooking, as a tea, or as a supplement.

M - COMPREHENSIVE GUIDE TO NATURAL REMEDIES FOR EVERYDAY HEALTH CONCERNS

MALARIA

Malaria, a life-threatening disease transmitted by mosquitoes, requires prompt medical treatment. Some herbs are traditionally used to complement malaria treatment and alleviate symptoms.

- **Artemisia Annua (Sweet Wormwood):** The source of artemisinin, used in modern antimalarial drugs. Used in traditional medicine to treat malaria. Take as a tea or supplement under medical guidance.
- **Ginger:** Can help alleviate symptoms like nausea and improve appetite during recovery. Use fresh ingredients in cooking or as tea.

MEASLES

Measles is a highly contagious viral infection requiring medical attention. Herbal remedies focus on supporting the immune system and managing symptoms.

- **Echinacea:** Known for immune-boosting properties. It may help in reducing the duration of the illness. Take it as a tea or supplement.

- **Vitamin C-Rich Herbs (like Rosehips):** High in vitamin C, which can support the immune system. Consume as a tea or supplement.

MENOPAUSE

Menopause, marking the end of a woman's reproductive years, can come with symptoms like hot flashes and mood swings. Certain herbs can help manage these symptoms.

- **Black Cohosh:** Widely used for reducing menopausal symptoms, including hot flashes and mood disturbances. Take it as a supplement.
- **Red Clover:** Contains isoflavones and plant-based estrogens, which may help balance hormones and alleviate menopausal symptoms. Drink as tea or take as a supplement.

MENSTRUAL CRAMPS

Menstrual cramps can be alleviated using herbs with antispasmodic and anti-inflammatory properties.

- **Cramp Bark:** Specifically targets menstrual cramps. Take it as a tea or tincture.
- **Ginger:** Reduces the severity of pain and inflammation. Drink it as tea or use it fresh in cooking.

MIGRAINES

Migraines, severe headaches often accompanied by other symptoms, can be managed with herbs known for their pain-relieving properties.

- **Feverfew:** Known to reduce the frequency and severity of migraines. Take it as a supplement or tea.
- **Butterbur:** Can help reduce the frequency of migraine attacks. Use as a

supplement under medical guidance.

MUMPS

Mumps is a viral infection primarily affecting the salivary glands. Supportive herbal remedies focus on relieving symptoms and boosting immunity.

- **Echinacea:** Boosts the immune system. Take it as a tea or supplement.
- **Slippery Elm Throat Lozenges:** Can soothe a sore throat and pain from swollen glands. Use as directed.

Mental Well-being and Stress Relief

In today's fast-paced world, mental well-being and stress management are more important than ever. Herbal remedies have long been used to support mental health and alleviate stress.

Understanding Mental Well-being and Stress

Mental well-being encompasses emotional, psychological, and social wellness, affecting how we think, feel, and act. Stress, a common response to life's challenges, can impact mental health if not managed properly. Herbal remedies offer a natural way to enhance mental well-being and mitigate the effects of stress.

Herbal Remedies for Mental Well-being

St. John's Wort (Hypericum perforatum)

- **Uses:** Known for its antidepressant properties, it's used to treat mild to moderate depression.

- **How to Use:** Available in capsules, teas, and tinctures. It's important to note that St. John's Wort can interact with certain medications.

Valerian Root (Valeriana officinalis)

- **Uses:** Helps reduce anxiety and improve sleep quality.
- **How to Use:** Often taken as a supplement or tea before bedtime.

Lavender (Lavandula)

- **Uses:** Known for its calming effects, it helps reduce stress and anxiety.
- **How to Use:** Used in aromatherapy, baths, or as an essential oil for massages.

Ashwagandha (Withania somnifera)

- **Uses:** An adaptogen that helps the body resist stressors, improves mood, and supports overall mental well-being.
- **How to Use:** Commonly taken as a supplement in powder or capsule form.

Herbal Remedies for Stress Relief

Lemon Balm (Melissa officinalis)

- **Uses:** Reduces stress and anxiety, promotes calmness, and improves sleep.
- **How to Use:** It can be taken as tea, in capsules, or used in aromatherapy.

Chamomile (Matricaria chamomilla)

- **Uses:** Soothes stress, calms nerves, and helps with sleep issues.
- **How to Use:** Commonly consumed as a relaxing tea.

Rhodiola Rosea

- **Uses:** An adaptogen that helps reduce fatigue and exhaustion in prolonged stressful situations.
- **How to Use:** Typically taken in supplement form.

Incorporating Herbs into Daily Life for Mental Well-being

Regular incorporation of these herbs into daily routines can significantly contribute to improved mental health and stress management. Whether starting the day with a cup of St. John's Wort tea, using lavender oil for relaxation, or taking an Ashwagandha supplement, these natural remedies can be powerful allies in maintaining mental balance.

Safety and Precautions

It's crucial to use these remedies responsibly. Some herbs can interact with medications or have side effects. Always consult with a healthcare professional, especially if you are under treatment for mental health issues.

N - COMPREHENSIVE GUIDE TO NATURAL REMEDIES FOR EVERYDAY HEALTH CONCERNS

NAIL FUNGUS

Nail fungus, or onychomycosis, is a common condition that causes discoloration, thickening, and separation of the nail from the nail bed. Herbal remedies can have antifungal properties that help treat nail fungus.

- **Tea Tree Oil:** Known for its antifungal and antiseptic properties. Apply diluted tea tree oil directly to the affected nail.
- **Oregano Oil:** Contains thymol, which has antifungal effects. Apply diluted oregano oil to the nail, but be cautious as it irritates the skin.

NAUSEA

Various factors, including motion sickness, pregnancy, or digestive issues, can cause nausea. Herbs can help soothe the stomach and reduce feelings of nausea.

- **Ginger:** Effective in treating nausea, including motion sickness and pregnancy-related nausea. Use fresh ginger in cooking, as a tea, or take ginger supplements.

- **Peppermint:** The aroma of peppermint can relieve nausea. Use peppermint oil for aromatherapy or drink peppermint tea.

NECK PAIN

Neck pain can arise from tension, poor posture, or other factors. Herbal remedies can help alleviate pain and reduce inflammation.

- **Turmeric:** Contains curcumin, which has anti-inflammatory properties. Use in cooking or as a supplement.
- **Willow Bark:** Often used for pain relief, as it contains salicin, a precursor to aspirin. Take it as a tea or supplement.

NIGHT SWEATS

Night sweats can occur due to hormonal changes, such as during menopause or from medical conditions. Certain herbs can help regulate the body's response to hormonal changes or help the body cool down.

- **Sage:** Has natural estrogenic properties and can help manage menopausal night sweats. Drink as a tea.
- **Black Cohosh:** Can reduce hot flashes and night sweats in menopausal women. Take it as a supplement.

O - COMPREHENSIVE GUIDE TO NATURAL REMEDIES FOR EVERYDAY HEALTH CONCERNS

OBESITY

Obesity, characterized by excessive body fat, is a risk factor for various health conditions. Herbal remedies can support weight loss by enhancing metabolism, reducing appetite, or improving digestion.

- **Green Tea:** Green Tea contains catechins and caffeine, which can aid in weight loss by enhancing metabolism. Drink green tea regularly.
- **Garcinia Cambogia:** A fruit extract believed to suppress appetite and inhibit fat production. Use as directed in supplement form.

OSTEOARTHRITIS

Osteoarthritis involves the degeneration of joint cartilage, leading to pain and stiffness. Herbs with anti-inflammatory and analgesic properties can help manage symptoms.

- **Turmeric:** The curcumin in turmeric is a potent anti-inflammatory agent. Use in cooking or as a supplement, often combined with black pepper to enhance absorption.

- **Boswellia:** Also known as Indian frankincense, it has anti-inflammatory effects that benefit osteoarthritis. Available as a supplement.

OSTEOPOROSIS

Osteoporosis is characterized by weakened bones that are more susceptible to fractures. Herbs rich in calcium and other bone-supporting nutrients can be beneficial.

- **Horsetail:** It contains silica, a mineral important for bone health. Use as a tea or supplement.
- **Red Clover:** Rich in isoflavones, which may positively affect bone density. Drink as a tea or take as a supplement.

OTITIS MEDIA (EAR INFECTION)

Otitis media, a middle ear infection, often requires medical treatment. Herbal remedies can be used to alleviate pain and inflammation.

- **Garlic Oil:** Known for its antimicrobial properties. Apply warm garlic oil drops into the ear, but avoid if the eardrum is perforated.
- **Mullein Ear Drops:** Often combined with garlic oil, mullein can reduce inflammation. Use as ear drops, ensuring there's no eardrum perforation.

P - COMPREHENSIVE GUIDE TO NATURAL REMEDIES FOR EVERYDAY HEALTH CONCERNS

PAIN

Pain can be acute or chronic and stems from various causes. Herbs with analgesic and anti-inflammatory properties can help manage pain.

- **Ginger:** Reduces inflammation and can alleviate pain. Use in cooking, as a tea, or as a supplement.
- **Capsaicin (from Cayenne Peppers):** Helps reduce pain signals when applied topically. Use as a cream or ointment.

PANIC DISORDER

Panic disorder involves sudden episodes of intense fear. Herbs with calming and anxiolytic properties can help manage symptoms.

- **Valerian Root:** Acts as a natural sedative, reducing anxiety and promoting relaxation. Take it as a tea or supplement.
- **Passionflower:** Known for its calming effects, it can help alleviate symptoms of panic attacks. Use as a tea or tincture.

PARKINSON'S DISEASE

Parkinson's disease affects movement, and while herbs cannot cure it, they can help manage some symptoms and support overall health.

- **Mucuna Pruriens (Velvet Bean):** Contains levodopa, a precursor to dopamine, and may help manage symptoms. Use under medical guidance.
- **Ginkgo Biloba** May help with cognitive symptoms. Take it as a supplement.

PEPTIC ULCER DISEASE

Peptic ulcers are sores in the lining of the stomach or small intestine. Herbs that provide mucosal protection and reduce acidity can be helpful.

- **Licorice Root:** Stimulates mucosal production, protecting the lining of the stomach. Use DGL (deglycyrrhizinated licorice) to avoid side effects.
- **Slippery Elm:** Forms a soothing layer over the ulcer. Drink as a tea or use as a supplement.

PINK EYE (Conjunctivitis)

Pink eye, an inflammation of the conjunctiva, often requires medical treatment. Mild herbal remedies can provide relief from symptoms.

- **Chamomile:** Anti-inflammatory properties can soothe irritation. Use as a warm compress (ensure it's sterile).
- **Eyebright:** Traditionally used for eye irritations. Use as a sterile eye wash or compress.

PNEUMONIA

Pneumonia, an infection of the lungs, requires medical attention. Herbs can support the immune system and help in recovery.

- **Echinacea:** Boosts the immune system. Take it as a tea or supplement.
- **Thyme:** Has antimicrobial properties and can support respiratory health. Drink as a tea.

POLYCYSTIC OVARY SYNDROME (PCOS)

PCOS is a hormonal disorder causing enlarged ovaries with cysts. Herbs that regulate hormones and improve insulin sensitivity can be beneficial.

- **Spearmint tea may** help reduce androgen levels.
- **Cinnamon:** Can improve insulin sensitivity. Use in cooking or as a supplement.

POST-TRAUMATIC STRESS DISORDER (PTSD)

PTSD is a mental health condition triggered by a traumatic event. Herbs with calming effects can support coping mechanisms.

- **Ashwagandha:** An adaptogen that helps the body resist stressors. Take it as a supplement.
- **Lavender:** Known for its calming effects. Use in aromatherapy or as a tea.

PREGNANCY-RELATED CONDITIONS

Herbal remedies for pregnancy-related conditions like morning sickness or gestational diabetes should be used with extreme caution and under medical supervision.

- **Ginger:** Can alleviate morning sickness. Use in moderation as a tea or fresh ginger.
- **Raspberry Leaf:** Often used in the third trimester to tone the uterus for labor. Drink as a tea.

PREMENSTRUAL SYNDROME (PMS)

PMS encompasses various symptoms before menstruation. Herbs can help alleviate these symptoms.

- **Chasteberry (Vitex):** Known to help balance hormones and relieve PMS symptoms. Take it as a supplement.
- **Dandelion:** Can help reduce bloating. Drink as a tea.

PROSTATE PROBLEMS

Herbal remedies can support prostate health and alleviate symptoms of conditions like benign prostatic hyperplasia (BPH).

- **Saw Palmetto:** Commonly used for BPH symptoms. Take it as a supplement.
- **Pygeum:** African plum tree bark extract known for its benefits in prostate health. Take it as a supplement.

R - COMPREHENSIVE GUIDE TO NATURAL REMEDIES FOR EVERYDAY HEALTH CONCERNS

REACTIVE ARTHRITIS

Reactive arthritis is a type of arthritis that occurs as a reaction to an infection in another part of the body. Herbal remedies can help manage symptoms like joint pain and inflammation.

- **Turmeric:** It contains curcumin, a potent anti-inflammatory compound. Use in cooking or as a supplement.
- **Ginger is also** anti-inflammatory and can help reduce joint pain. Use fresh in cooking, as a tea, or as a supplement.

REFLUX ESOPHAGITIS

Reflux esophagitis is inflammation of the oesophagus caused by acid reflux. Herbs that soothe the digestive tract and reduce acidity can provide relief.

- **Slippery Elm:** Forms a soothing gel that coats the lining of the oesophagus. Consume as a tea or in capsules.
- **Marshmallow Root:** Soothes the inflamed oesophagus and protects from stomach acid. Use as a tea or supplement.

RHEUMATOID ARTHRITIS

Rheumatoid arthritis is an autoimmune disease that causes chronic inflammation of the joints. Herbs with anti-inflammatory and immune-modulating properties can help manage symptoms.

- **Boswellia:** Known for its anti-inflammatory properties. Take it as a supplement.
- **Green Tea:** Green Tea contains polyphenols, which may help reduce inflammation and support immune function. Drink regularly as a tea.

RINGWORM

Ringworm is a fungal infection of the skin. Herbal remedies with antifungal properties can be used topically to treat the infection.

- **Tea Tree Oil:** Has strong antifungal properties. Apply diluted tea tree oil to the affected area.
- **Garlic:** Allicin in garlic is antifungal. Apply garlic paste to the affected area or use diluted garlic oil.

Respiratory Issues

Respiratory health is vital for overall well-being, and throughout history, various cultures have turned to herbal remedies to treat common respiratory ailments.

Understanding Respiratory Health

The respiratory system, crucial for breathing, is often susceptible to infections and allergies. Conditions like the common cold, cough, bronchitis, asthma, and sinusitis are prevalent. While conventional medicine offers relief, herbal remedies can be effective alternatives or complements, often with fewer side effects.

Herbal Remedies for Respiratory Conditions

Eucalyptus (Eucalyptus globulus)

- **Uses:** Relieves coughs and decongests the chest. Its main component, eucalyptol, helps loosen phlegm.
- **How to Use:** Inhaled via steam or used in chest rubs. Eucalyptus oil should not be ingested.

Mullein (Verbascum thapsus)

- **Uses:** Soothes the respiratory tract and is used for dry coughs and bronchial irritations.
- **How to Use:** Consumed as tea or used in tinctures. Inhalation of its steam is also beneficial.

Licorice Root (Glycyrrhiza glabra)

- **Uses:** Acts as an expectorant, soothing the throat and easing congestion.
- **How to Use:** Taken as a tea, chewed on as a stick, or used in cough syrups.

Thyme (Thymus vulgaris)

- **Uses:** Has antibacterial and antispasmodic properties, making it effective for coughs and bronchitis.
- **How to Use:** Consumed as tea or used in cooking. Thyme oil can also be diluted and applied topically.

Peppermint (Mentha piperita)

- **Uses:** Menthol in peppermint helps clear the nasal passage and relieves throat irritation.

- **How to Use:** Peppermint tea is common, as are tablets and inhalants.

Integrating Herbs into Respiratory Care

These herbs can be incorporated into daily routines to support respiratory health, especially during cold and flu season. Drinking herbal teas or using aromatherapy with essential oils like eucalyptus or peppermint can be particularly beneficial.

Safety and Precautions

It's essential to use these herbs judiciously, especially when dealing with essential oils, which can be potent. Individuals with chronic respiratory conditions, pregnant women, or those on medication should consult healthcare professionals before using herbal remedies.

S - COMPREHENSIVE GUIDE TO NATURAL REMEDIES FOR EVERYDAY HEALTH CONCERNS

SCABIES

Scabies, a skin infestation caused by a mite, require medical treatment. Herbal remedies can soothe itching and aid skin healing.

- **Tea Tree Oil:** Has antiparasitic properties. Apply diluted tea tree oil to affected areas.
- **Neem:** Known for its antimicrobial and antiparasitic properties. Use neem oil or soap topically.

SINUSITIS

Sinusitis is inflammation of the sinuses, often leading to congestion, pain, and drainage. Herbs can help reduce inflammation and clear congestion.

- **Eucalyptus:** Inhaled eucalyptus steam can help clear sinus congestion.
- **Peppermint:** Its menthol content soothes congestion. Use in steam inhalation or drink as tea.

SKIN CANCER

Skin cancer requires conventional medical treatment. Some herbs may provide supportive care and protect skin health.

- **Green Tea:** Rich in antioxidants, topical application of green tea extract may provide protective effects against UV radiation.
- **Turmeric:** Its curcumin content might help in preventing skin damage. Use topically as a paste or orally as a supplement.

SLEEP APNEA

Sleep apnea is a serious sleep disorder that requires medical intervention. Herbs can support better sleep and reduce inflammation.

- **Valerian Root:** Promotes relaxation and better sleep quality. Take it as a tea or supplement.
- **Chamomile:** Helps with relaxation. Drink chamomile tea before bedtime.

SNORING

Snoring is often caused by airway obstruction. Some herbs can help in reducing inflammation and ease breathing.

- **Peppermint:** Anti-inflammatory properties can help reduce swelling in the nasal passages. Use peppermint oil in a diffuser.
- **Thyme:** Said to reduce snoring when used aromatically. Use in a diffuser or apply diluted oil topically.

SORE THROAT

A sore throat can be soothed with herbs known for their anti-inflammatory and analgesic properties.

- **Licorice Root:** Soothes sore throat. Use as a gargle solution.
- **Slippery Elm:** Forms a soothing gel that coats the throat. Drink as a tea.

SPIDER BITES

Most spider bites are harmless, but some can be serious. Herbal remedies can reduce pain and swelling.

- **Aloe Vera:** Soothes the skin and reduces inflammation. Apply aloe gel to the bite.
- **Baking Soda:** Not an herb, but a paste made with baking soda and water can relieve itching and swelling.

SPRAINS AND STRAINS

Sprains and strains involve injury to ligaments and muscles. Herbs can help reduce swelling and speed up healing.

- **Arnica:** Reduces pain and swelling. Use as a cream or gel.
- **Comfrey:** Known for aiding in the healing of sprains. Apply as a cream or poultice, but not on broken skin.

SEXUALLY TRANSMITTED INFECTIONS (STIs)

STIs like gonorrhea and syphilis require medical treatment. Some herbs can support immune function and complement conventional treatments.

- **Goldenseal:** Has antimicrobial properties. Take it as a supplement or tea.

- **Echinacea:** Boosts immune function. Take it as a tea or supplement.

STOMACH FLU

Stomach flu, or viral gastroenteritis, causes diarrhea and vomiting. Herbs can help in rehydration and soothing the digestive tract.

- **Ginger:** Reduces nausea and vomiting. Drink as a tea.
- **Peppermint:** Relieves abdominal pain. Drink as a tea.

STRESS

Chronic stress impacts overall health. Herbs with calming and adaptogenic properties can help manage stress.

- **Ashwagandha:** An adaptogen that helps the body resist stressors. Take it as a supplement.
- **Holy Basil (Tulsi):** Reduces stress and anxiety. Drink as a tea.

STROKE

A stroke is a medical emergency requiring immediate attention. Post-stroke, certain herbs may aid in recovery and prevent recurrence.

- **Ginkgo Biloba** May improve cognitive function and circulation post-stroke. Take it as a supplement.
- **Garlic:** Helps in preventing blood clots. Include in diet or take as a supplement.

SUBSTANCE ABUSE

Substance abuse is a complex condition requiring specialized treatment. Some herbs can support detoxification and recovery.

- **Milk Thistle:** Supports liver detoxification. Take it as a supplement.
- **Kudzu Root:** May reduce cravings for alcohol. Use as directed in supplement form.

SUNBURN

Sunburn is skin damage caused by UV radiation. Soothing herbs can alleviate pain and promote healing.

- **Aloe Vera:** Cools and soothes sunburned skin. Apply aloe vera gel to affected areas.
- **Green Tea:** Antioxidants in green tea can help heal sunburn. Apply cooled green tea bags to the skin.

Skin and Hair Care

In the pursuit of natural beauty and wellness, the role of herbal remedies in skin and hair care is significant.

Understanding the Importance of Natural Care

Skin and hair are not just external beauty features but are also indicators of overall health. They constantly face environmental stressors, chemicals, and internal health fluctuations. Herbal remedies, with their natural properties, offer a gentler and often effective alternative to chemical-based products.

Herbal Remedies for Skin Care

Aloe Vera (Aloe barbadensis miller)

- **Uses:** Moisturizes skin, heals sunburns, and treats acne.
- **How to Use:** Apply the gel directly from the plant or use natural aloe vera products.

Calendula (Calendula officinalis)

- **Uses:** Soothes irritated skin, heals wounds, and reduces inflammation.
- **How to Use:** Used in creams, ointments, or infusions for topical application.

Tea Tree Oil (Melaleuca alternifolia)

- **Uses:** Effective against acne, dandruff, and skin infections due to its antimicrobial properties.
- **How to Use:** Dilute with a carrier oil for topical application or use in shampoos and cleansers.

Chamomile (Matricaria chamomilla)

- **Uses:** Calms sensitive skin, reduces redness and has anti-inflammatory properties.
- **How to Use:** Use in facial steams, teas, or skincare products for its soothing effect.

Herbal Remedies for Hair Care

Rosemary (Rosmarinus officinalis)

- **Uses:** Stimulates hair growth, boosts scalp circulation, and reduces

dandruff.
- **How to Use:** Use rosemary oil in scalp massages or add rosemary leaves to hair rinses.

Lavender (Lavandula)

- **Uses:** Promotes hair growth, prevents hair loss, and has a calming effect on the scalp.
- **How to Use:** Add lavender oil to shampoo conditioners or use in scalp massages.

Nettle (Urtica dioica)

- **Uses:** Rich in nutrients that nourish hair follicles, reduce hair loss, and improve scalp health.
- **How to Use:** Use nettle infusions as a hair rinse or include them in hair care formulations.

Incorporating Herbal Remedies in Daily Regimens

Incorporating these herbs into daily skin and hair care routines can be simple yet effective. Making herbal infusions for hair rinses, using oils for scalp massages, or applying herbal-based creams and ointments can provide natural, nourishing care.

Safety and Sensitivity

As with all herbal remedies, awareness of potential allergies and skin sensitivities is crucial, conducting patch tests and consulting with a dermatologist or trichologist, especially in cases of severe skin or scalp conditions, is advisable.

T - COMPREHENSIVE GUIDE TO NATURAL REMEDIES FOR EVERYDAY HEALTH CONCERNS

TENDINITIS

Tendinitis is the inflammation of a tendon, often causing pain and tenderness near joints. Herbal remedies can help reduce inflammation and alleviate pain.

- **Turmeric:** Contains curcumin, which has potent anti-inflammatory effects. Use in cooking or as a supplement.
- **Bromelain:** An enzyme found in pineapples, known for its anti-inflammatory properties. Take as a supplement, often combined with turmeric, for enhanced effect.

TENNIS ELBOW

Tennis elbow is a type of tendinitis that causes pain in the elbow and arm. Herbs with anti-inflammatory and analgesic properties can help manage symptoms.

- **Arnica:** Known for reducing pain and inflammation. Use topically as a cream or gel.
- **White Willow Bark:** Natural aspirin-like effects can help alleviate pain.

Take it as a tea or supplement.

TESTICULAR CANCER

Testicular cancer requires conventional medical treatment. Certain herbs may support overall health and complement cancer treatments.

- **Green Tea:** High in antioxidants, which may have cancer-fighting properties. Drink as a tea.
- **Astragalus:** Used in traditional medicine to support immune function, which can be beneficial during cancer treatments. Take it as a supplement or tea.

TETANUS

Tetanus is a serious bacterial infection that affects the nervous system and requires immediate medical treatment. Post-treatment, some herbs can support recovery.

- **Echinacea:** Boosts the immune system. Take it as a tea or supplement.
- **Goldenseal:** Has antimicrobial properties. Use as a supplement under medical guidance.

TONSILLITIS

Tonsillitis, inflammation of the tonsils, can be soothed with herbs known for their anti-inflammatory and antimicrobial properties.

- **Slippery Elm:** Soothes inflamed throat tissues. Drink as a tea or use in tablets.
- **Thyme:** Antimicrobial properties can help fight infection. Drink as a tea or use as a gargle.

TRAUMATIC BRAIN INJURY (TBI)

TBI requires specialized medical treatment. Post-injury, certain herbs may support brain health and recovery.

- **Ginkgo Biloba** May improve cognitive function after a brain injury. Take it as a supplement.
- **Omega-3 Fatty Acids (from Fish Oil):** Supports brain health. Use fish oil supplements.

TUBERCULOSIS (TB)

Tuberculosis is a serious bacterial infection affecting the lungs and requires medical treatment. Herbs can support the immune system and complement TB treatment.

- **Astragalus:** Enhances immune response. Use as a supplement or tea.
- **Garlic:** Has natural antimicrobial properties. Include fresh garlic in your diet, or take it as a supplement.

U - COMPREHENSIVE GUIDE TO NATURAL REMEDIES FOR EVERYDAY HEALTH CONCERNS

ULCERATIVE COLITIS

Ulcerative colitis is a chronic inflammatory bowel disease affecting the colon and rectum. Herbal remedies can help manage inflammation and soothe the digestive tract.

- **Aloe Vera:** Known for its anti-inflammatory and healing properties. Drink aloe vera juice to soothe the digestive tract.
- **Turmeric:** Contains curcumin, which can reduce inflammation. Use in cooking or take as a supplement with black pepper for better absorption.

URINARY INCONTINENCE

Urinary incontinence, the loss of bladder control, can be managed with herbs that strengthen the urinary tract and bladder.

- **Horsetail:** Acts as a natural diuretic and toning agent for the bladder. Take it as a tea or supplement.
- **Gosha-jinki-gan:** A traditional Japanese herbal remedy, has shown benefits in reducing urinary incontinence. Use under guidance from a

qualified practitioner.

URINARY TRACT INFECTIONS (UTIs)

UTIs are typically caused by bacteria and often require antibiotics. Herbs can be used to alleviate symptoms and prevent recurrence.

- **Cranberry:** Helps prevent bacteria from adhering to the urinary tract walls. Drink unsweetened cranberry juice or take it as a supplement.
- **D-Mannose:** A sugar that can help prevent certain types of bacteria from sticking to the walls of the urinary tract. Take it as a supplement.

V - COMPREHENSIVE GUIDE TO NATURAL REMEDIES FOR EVERYDAY HEALTH CONCERNS

VARICOSE VEINS

Varicose veins are enlarged, twisted veins often found in the legs. Herbal remedies can support circulation and reduce inflammation.

- **Horse Chestnut:** Known to strengthen blood vessel walls and reduce symptoms of varicose veins. Available as a supplement.
- **Witch Hazel:** Applied topically, it can reduce swelling and discomfort associated with varicose veins. Use as a compress or in creams.

VERTIGO

Vertigo is a sensation of spinning or losing balance. Herbal treatments focus on improving inner ear health and reducing symptoms.

- **Ginger:** Can help reduce dizziness and nausea associated with vertigo. Take it as a tea or supplement.
- **Ginkgo Biloba:** Improves blood flow to the brain and may help with vertigo symptoms. Take it as a supplement.

VIRAL HEPATITIS

Viral hepatitis, an inflammation of the liver, requires medical treatment. Certain herbs can support liver function and complement conventional treatments.

- **Milk Thistle:** Supports liver health and is commonly used by those with liver conditions. Take it as a supplement.
- **Dandelion:** Acts as a liver tonic and may help improve liver function. Drink as a tea or use as a supplement.

VITAMIN DEFICIENCIES

Vitamin deficiencies should be addressed primarily through diet or supplements, but certain herbs can also provide vitamins.

- **Nettle:** High in vitamins A, C, and K, as well as minerals like iron and calcium. Use as a tea or cooked like spinach.
- **Parsley:** Rich in vitamins A, C, and K. Incorporate fresh parsley into your diet regularly.

W - COMPREHENSIVE GUIDE TO NATURAL REMEDIES FOR EVERYDAY HEALTH CONCERNS

WHOOPING COUGH (Pertussis)

Whooping cough, or pertussis, is a highly contagious respiratory tract infection marked by severe coughing. It can be particularly dangerous for infants and young children. While vaccination and medical treatment are key in managing whooping cough, some herbal remedies can help alleviate symptoms and support recovery.

- **Thyme:** Known for its antimicrobial and expectorant properties, thyme can help loosen phlegm and reduce coughing. Use as a tea or inhalant.
- **Honey:** While not an herb, honey (especially Manuka honey) has antibacterial properties and can soothe the throat, reducing coughing fits. It can be added to herbal teas or taken alone. Note: Honey should not be given to children under one-year-old due to the risk of botulism.
- **Marshmallow Root:** Has soothing properties that can relieve irritation in the throat and dry cough. Use as a tea or in a syrup form.
- **Licorice Root:** Soothes the throat and helps reduce the severity of cough. Take it as tea or use it in a syrup form. Using licorice root judiciously is important, as excessive consumption can lead to adverse side effects.

Supportive Care:

- Hydration: Drinking fluids, such as water and herbal teas, can help keep the throat moist and reduce irritation.
- Humidification: A humidifier in the bedroom can help ease breathing and coughing, especially at night.

Caution and Professional Care:

- Whooping cough can be serious, especially in young children and older people. It is crucial to follow professional medical advice and treatment plans.
- Pregnant women, infants, and people with chronic health conditions should exercise caution and consult with healthcare professionals before using any herbal remedies.

Herbal remedies can provide symptomatic relief for whooping cough, but they should be used as a complement to, not a substitute for, conventional medical treatment, including antibiotics and supportive care.

X - COMPREHENSIVE GUIDE TO NATURAL REMEDIES FOR EVERYDAY HEALTH CONCERNS

XEROSTOMIA (Dry Mouth)

Xerostomia, commonly known as dry mouth, is a condition where the salivary glands in your mouth don't produce enough saliva. This condition can be uncomfortable, causing difficulty tasting, chewing, swallowing, and speaking. While it's often a side effect of medication or a symptom of certain medical conditions, some herbal remedies can help stimulate saliva production and provide relief.

- **Ginger:** Known for its stimulating properties, ginger can encourage saliva production. Chew on a piece of fresh ginger, or drink ginger tea.
- **Fennel Seeds:** These have a similar stimulating effect on saliva production. Chew on fennel seeds throughout the day or drink fennel tea.
- **Aloe Vera Juice:** It helps to moisturize and soothe the dry tissues in the mouth. Drink aloe vera juice or rinse your mouth with it.
- **Green Tea:** Green Tea contains polyphenols that can help alleviate dry mouth. Drink green tea regularly. Ensure it is caffeine-free if caffeine exacerbates your dry mouth.
- **Slippery Elm:** Forms a mucilage that can coat and soothe the mouth, relieving dryness. Use as a tablet or drink as a tea.

Supportive Practices:

- Stay Hydrated: Drinking plenty of water throughout the day helps keep the mouth moist.
- Avoid Mouthwashes Containing Alcohol, As they can be drying.
- Humidify Your Environment: A humidifier, especially at night, can add moisture to the air and help relieve symptoms.

Caution:

- If xerostomia is a side effect of medication, do not discontinue or adjust your medication without consulting a healthcare professional.
- A healthcare provider should evaluate persistent dry mouth as it can be a sign of underlying health issues and lead to complications like tooth decay and gum disease.

Herbal remedies for xerostomia offer a natural way to alleviate discomfort, but addressing the condition's underlying cause is important. Always consult a healthcare provider for a comprehensive approach to treatment, especially if the condition persists or is accompanied by other symptoms.

Y - COMPREHENSIVE GUIDE TO NATURAL REMEDIES FOR EVERYDAY HEALTH CONCERNS

YELLOW FEVER

Yellow fever is a serious viral infection transmitted by mosquitoes, predominantly in parts of Africa and South America. It's characterized by fever, jaundice, muscle pain, and nausea. Yellow fever requires immediate medical attention, and an effective vaccine is available for its prevention.

While herbal remedies cannot cure yellow fever, they can be used to alleviate some symptoms under medical supervision:

- **Milk Thistle:** Supports liver function, which can be beneficial because yellow fever often affects the liver. Available as a supplement.
- **Dandelion:** Acts as a liver tonic and may help with symptoms of jaundice. Drink as a tea or use as a supplement.

Note: These herbs do not replace professional medical treatment and vaccination. If yellow fever is suspected, seek immediate medical attention.

YEAST INFECTIONS

Yeast infections are typically caused by the fungus Candida and can occur in various parts of the body, such as the mouth, throat, gut, and vagina. Herbal remedies with antifungal properties can be used to complement medical treatment.

- **Garlic:** Has natural antifungal properties. It can be included in the diet or taken as a supplement.
- **Tea Tree Oil:** For vaginal yeast infections, diluted tea tree oil can be applied topically. It should be used cautiously, as it can irritate sensitive skin.
- **Coconut Oil:** Contains caprylic acid, known for its antifungal properties. It can be applied topically or used in cooking.
- **Oregano Oil:** Has strong antifungal effects. Use as a supplement or apply diluted oregano oil topically.

Note: While these remedies can help manage yeast infection symptoms, they should not replace medical treatment, especially in persistent or severe cases. Consulting a healthcare provider for accurate diagnosis and appropriate treatment is important. Additionally, always conduct a patch test for topical applications to check for allergic reactions.

Z - COMPREHENSIVE GUIDE TO NATURAL REMEDIES FOR EVERYDAY HEALTH CONCERNS

ZIKA VIRUS

Zika virus is a mosquito-borne virus that can cause flu-like symptoms and is particularly concerning for pregnant women due to its potential to cause congenital disabilities. There is no specific treatment for Zika virus, and care is generally supportive.

Herbal remedies may help alleviate some symptoms of Zika virus, but they cannot cure the infection:

- **Echinacea:** Known for its immune-boosting properties, it may help the body fight viral infections. Take it as a tea or supplement.
- **Goldenseal:** Has antiviral and antibacterial properties. Use as a supplement or tea, but only for short-term use.

Important: Preventing mosquito bites remains crucial in areas where Zika virus is prevalent. Pregnant women or those planning pregnancy should follow medical advice, especially regarding travel to affected areas. Always consult a healthcare provider for proper guidance.

ZOSTER (SHINGLES)

Shingles, caused by the reactivation of the chickenpox virus (varicella-zoster), are painful rashes that usually appear on one side of the body. While antiviral medication is the primary treatment, certain herbs can help alleviate symptoms:

- **Licorice Root:** Has antiviral properties and may help reduce the severity of shingles. Apply topically as a gel or cream, or take as a tea or supplement.
- **Lemon Balm:** Known for its antiviral effects against herpes viruses, it can be applied topically to the rash to ease discomfort.
- **Calendula:** Helps in healing the skin and reducing inflammation. Use as a cream or ointment on the affected areas.

Note: Shingles can be serious, especially in older adults and people with weakened immune systems. It's important to start antiviral medications as soon as possible. Herbal remedies can provide symptomatic relief but should be used in conjunction with, not as a replacement for, conventional medical treatment. Consult a healthcare provider for a comprehensive treatment plan.

CONCLUSION

As we conclude our journey through "Herbal Solutions: The Comprehensive A-Z Guide to Natural Remedies for Everyday Health Concerns," we reflect on the invaluable insights gained into the world of herbal remedies. This guide has taught you about a vast array of herbs and their healing properties and has opened a path to a more natural, holistic approach to health and wellness.

Throughout this book, we've explored the intricate connections between nature and health, delving into how plants can offer gentle yet effective solutions to everyday ailments with their unique medicinal properties. From alleviating common cold symptoms with Echinacea to soothing digestive issues with peppermint, we've uncovered the potential of herbs to enhance well-being in a way that aligns with nature's rhythm.

"Herbal Solutions" stands as a testament to the power of natural healing. It encourages you to explore the therapeutic benefits of herbs, integrating them into your daily life as a proactive approach to health. The detailed profiles of each herb, coupled with practical advice on their use, have been designed to empower you, the reader, with the confidence to utilize these natural remedies safely and effectively.

Moreover, this book has highlighted the importance of understanding herbs - acknowledging their health benefits, limitations, and the necessity for responsible use.

As we close this comprehensive guide, we hope it serves as a reference and a catalyst for a deeper appreciation of herbal medicine. Whether you are dealing with minor health nuisances or seeking to maintain overall wellness, "Herbal Solutions" provides a roadmap to harnessing the natural efficacy of herbs.

In embracing the wisdom within these pages, you join a growing community of individuals turning to nature for answers to health concerns. This journey with herbs is about treating ailments and nurturing a lifelong relationship with the natural world, leading to a healthier, more balanced life.

SOURCES

https://www.medicalnewstoday.com/articles/322455#home-remedies

https://pharmeasy.in/blog/home-remedies-for-anaemia/

https://www.allinahealth.org/healthysetgo/heal/natural-remedies-for-ever
yday-illnesses

https://www.healthline.com/health/home-remedies

https://www.webmd.com/balance/ss/slideshow-home-remedies

https://stylecaster.com/beauty/beauty/349189/natural-remedies-for-every-
common-health-problem/

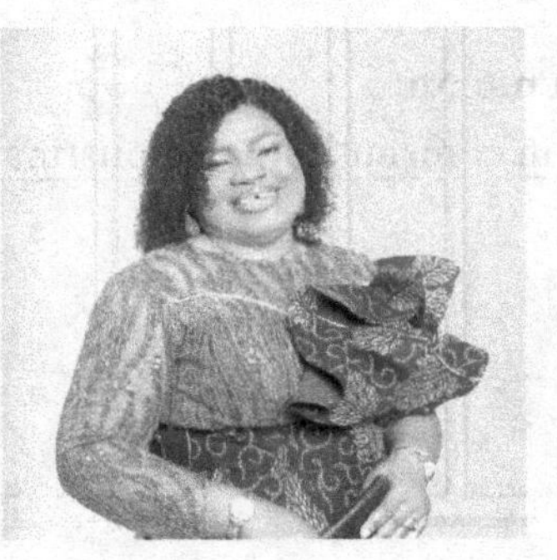

About the Author

Glorioustina Essia is a multifaceted professional whose expertise traverses the realms of technology, artificial intelligence, literature, and natural health. As a driving force in artificial intelligence, particularly in prompt engineering, she has established herself as a pioneer. Her proficiency extends to project management, network marketing, website development, and copywriting, showcasing a unique blend of technical understanding and creative flair.

A prolific author and publisher, Glorioustina's literary works span multiple genres, captivating a diverse audience with her narrative skill and inspiring a new generation of writers to unlock their creative potential. Her passion for storytelling matches her commitment to exploring and advocating for holistic health practices. Renowned in herbal medicine, she dedicates her life to studying and promoting natural health.

Glorioustina Essia's professional and personal journey is characterized by an unwavering dedication to her core strengths and a ceaseless pursuit of knowledge. Her zeal and expertise embody the limitless possibilities that arise from a commitment to innovation, quality, and a deep-seated passion for understanding the future of technology and the ancient wisdom of herbal medicine. Glorioustina is a testament to the power of interdisciplinary knowledge and its impact in a world where technology, literature, and natural health converge.

You can connect with me on:

🌐 https://www.amazon.com/author/glorioustina

Also by Glorioustina Essia

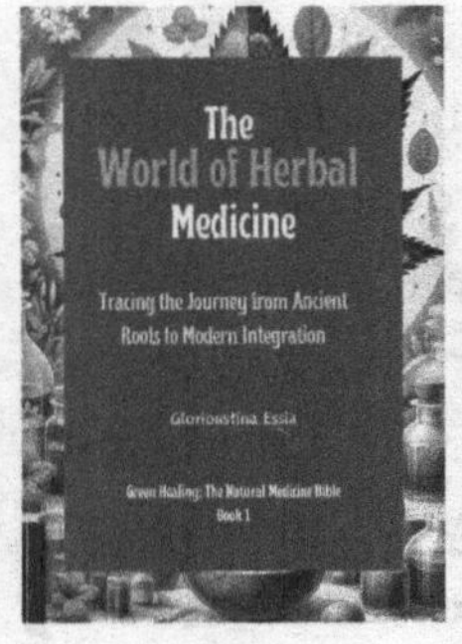

The World of Herbal Medicine

In an era where the rush of modern medicine often overshadows the pursuit of holistic health, the timeless wisdom of herbal remedies remains largely untapped. Do you find yourself seeking a more natural approach to health and wellness yet still determining where to begin or how to integrate these practices with modern healthcare?

Embark on a transformative journey with Book 1 of "Green Healing: The Natural Medicine Bible": "The World of Herbal Medicine." This enlightening volume takes you through the ancient pathways to the modern integration of herbal healing. Discover herbal medicine's rich history and evolution across different cultures, including the profound insights of Traditional Chinese Medicine, Ayurveda, and indigenous practices. Unravel how herbalism has evolved through historical epochs and how it beautifully intersects with modern medical practices today.

Embrace the journey to holistic health – add this captivating volume to your collection and begin exploring the world of herbal medicine today

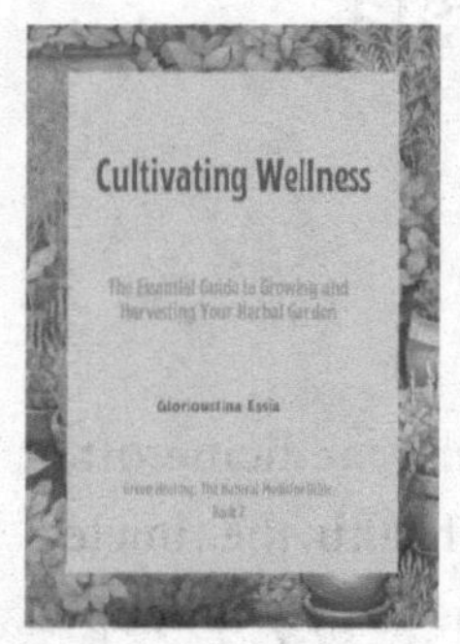

Cultivating Wellness

This guide is your gateway to mastering the art of herb gardening, offering practical advice for cultivating various medicinal and culinary herbs. From sustainable techniques to harvesting and preservation methods, each chapter brims with expert knowledge tailored to beginners and experienced gardeners. Learn to navigate common challenges in herb gardening and create specialized gardens for your health and culinary needs. Beyond gardening tips, this book inspires a deeper connection with nature and a commitment to a holistic lifestyle. Embrace the journey of nurturing not just a garden but a healthier, more harmonious way of life with "Cultivating Wellness."

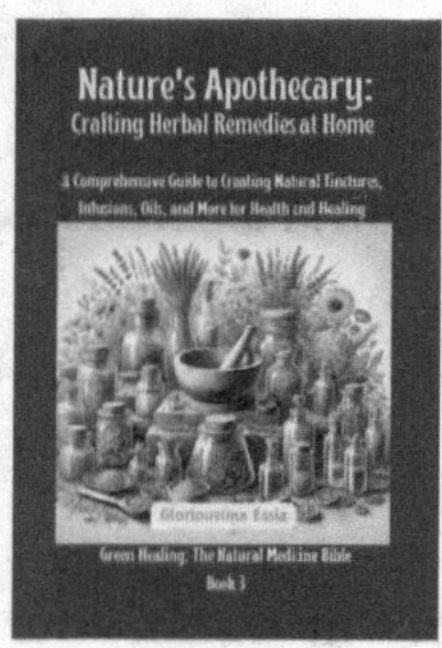

Nature's Apothecary

This comprehensive guide demystifies making your natural tinctures, infusions, oils, and more. It provides step-by-step instructions and detailed information on various herbs and their medicinal properties, empowering you to create effective, natural remedies in your kitchen.

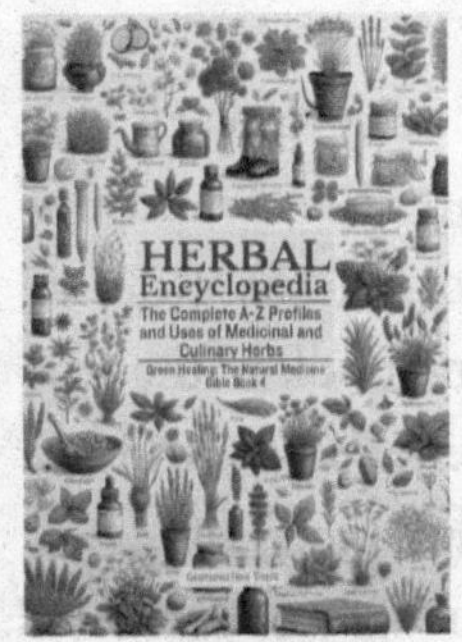

Herbal Encyclopedia

Embark on a journey through nature's apothecary with "Herbal Encyclopedia: The Complete A-Z Profiles and Uses of Medicinal and Culinary Herbs." This guide unravels the secrets of herbs, from age-old medicinal uses to enhancing culinary delights. Each page introduces you to a new herb, revealing its history, health benefits, and how it can be incorporated into your daily life. Whether you're a budding herbalist or a seasoned enthusiast, this encyclopedia offers easy-to-understand profiles, practical tips, and a connection to the ancient art of herbal healing.

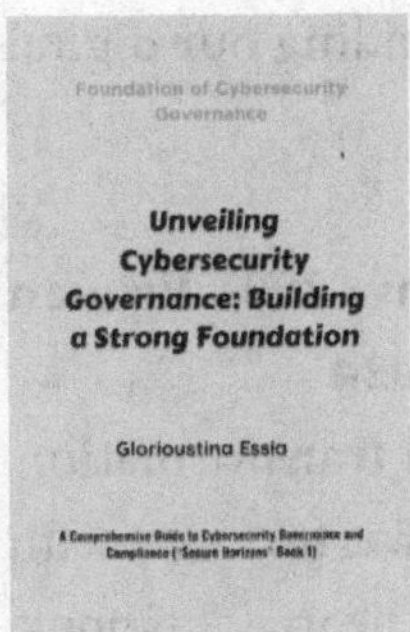

Unveiling Cybersecurity Governance

In the ever-expanding digital landscape, safeguarding sensitive information and maintaining robust cybersecurity practices have become paramount. "Unveiling Cybersecurity Governance: Building a Strong Foundation" is a comprehensive guide that delves into cybersecurity governance's core principles and components, equipping readers with the knowledge and tools to establish a secure digital environment.

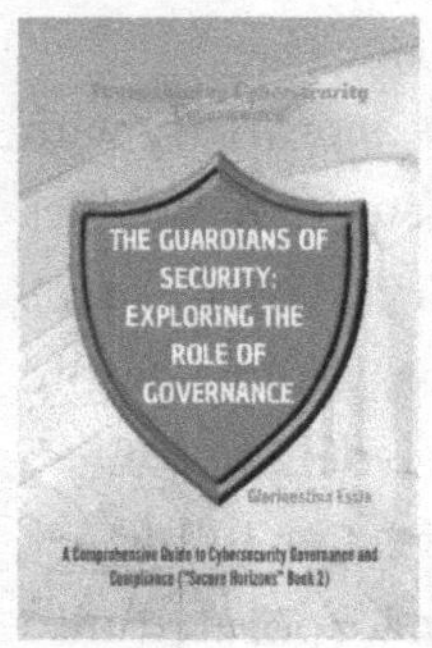

THE GUARDIANS OF SECURITY

Step into a world where cybersecurity governance catalyzes a secure future. Explore the realms of "The Guardians of Security: Exploring the Role of Governance," the much-awaited second book in the epic series "Secure Horizons: A Comprehensive Guide to Cybersecurity Governance and Compliance."

As you read each page of "The Guardians of Security," prepare to be enchanted by the author's remarkable storytelling ability. This book presents a vivid picture of the complicated landscape of cybersecurity governance with a seamless blend of real-world experiences, cutting-edge research, and visionary concepts. Immerse yourself in an exciting story that uncovers the brains and souls of people dedicated to defending our digital borders.

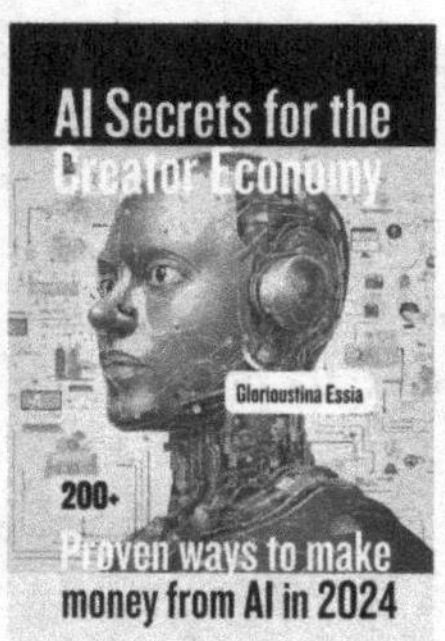

AI Secrets for the Creator Economy: 200+ Proven ways to make money from AI in 2024

In a world driven by innovation and transformation, the Creator Economy emerges as a powerful force, with Artificial Intelligence (AI) at its beating heart. This book, "AI Secrets for the Creator Economy: 200+ Proven Ways to Make Money from AI in 2024 and Beyond," is more than just a book; it's your key to unlocking the incredible synergy between AI and creativity, opening the door to a wealth of opportunities for those who are willing to seize them.